# The
# Moveme
## Book

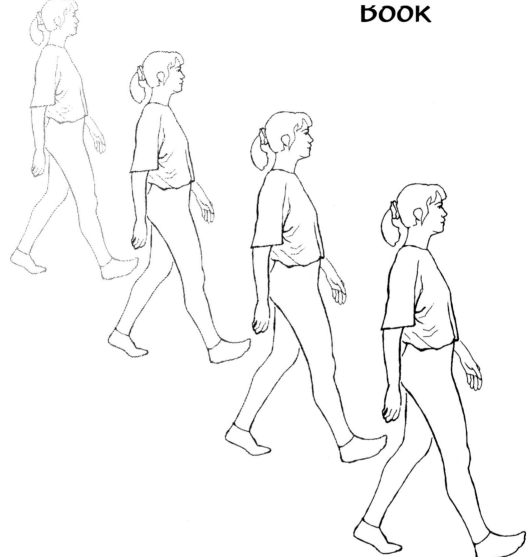

# Ken Thompson

bibliotek books

# Dedication

To the many teachers and guides I have been fortunate to meet and learn from, I would like to say a big 'thank you'. It would be impossible for me to list you all but I would like to express my gratitude to ten people who, at a certain point in my life, have had a strong influence on me and have perhaps been instrumental in changing my life's course.

To Albert Drew for stimulating my interest in health and fitness, and to Derek Johnson for his encouraging football management.

To Chris Stevens for his enthusiasm, and for introducing me to the Alexander Technique, and to Paul Collins for superb lessons; to Walter Carrington for his infinite patience and understanding, and for a training of which F. M. Alexander would wholeheartedly have approved.

To J. Krishnamurti and the Talks at Brockwood Park, which marked a turning point in my thinking.

To Wilfred Clark for his dedication and a dream of Yoga Unity throughout the UK; and to Swami Sivananda of Rishikesh for sending such wonderful, inspired teachers around the world.

To Gordon Higginson for his positive teaching, and for finding life in death; and finally, to my wife, Angela, for her support and encouragement through good and bad times.

IN THE SILENCE OF KNOWING WE ARE ALL ONE.
Ken Thompson

Published in 1996 by
Bibliotek Books
19 Warwick Road,
Stafford, UK
ISBN I 873017 10 3

# Contents

# Introduction

## How this book came to be written

In the summer of 1993 John and Mary Salisbury and I got together to discuss the possibility of a movement book.

For over 20 years I have devoted a great deal of interest to the problem of poor co-ordination among students at the yoga classes that I have been running. I know that, in learning new skills, the body tends to adapt itself to achieve the results we want. But the adaptations that it makes are not always constructive and indeed, in a good many cases, are detrimental, in the long run, to the psychophysical system.

How can this be avoided? Well, the first step is to help people become aware that they are not always doing exactly what they think they are doing! Then, if possible, to guide them towards improving the situation. This is how 'co-ordination movements' came into being: they are a simple, but extremely efficient means of expanding awareness into body movements.

## This book is about improving co-ordination

It must be emphasised that the movements in this book are not designed to develop strength or stamina, but to improve co-ordination.

In response to the considerable current interest in taking more personal responsibility for one's health, many books are now available which stress the importance of strength, stamina and mobility. These qualities, obviously, are important. But, however strong, supple and energetic you are, as long as you are poorly co-ordinated, you will not function as well as you could. This is an undisputed fact!

Most people are not well co-ordinated, a fact which is fairly easy to demonstrate. It is apparent to many people when they come to engage in a sport or learn a new skill - but less noticeable in everyday activities. It may be that we move less well now than we did when we lived closer to nature. Whatever the reason, the important thing now is, what can we do for ourselves to remedy the situation?

The movements selected here have been throughly tested by myself and many of my students over many years, and have proved successful. Do not let their simplicity deceive you into underestimating their effectiveness!They work at a subtle level, incorporating the power of thought into movement. This power has been recognised for hundreds of years in many physical training systems, which have always understood that you must 'follow the movement with your mind' to get the best results.

These movements, synchronised with your own breathing rhythm, help you to focus your mind and monitor your performance, bringing mind and body into harmony.

## Maintaining the working integrity of yourself

By the 'working integrity of yourself' I mean all the ongoing vital systems that keep you alive and enable you to move: your breathing, circulation, digestion, and the flow of nervous energy, neuromuscular connections, etc.

The breathing rhythm is chosen to govern the pace of the movements in this book because it provides such an instant and reliable feedback device, giving you notice of any lowering of your working integrity. For example, you must have noticed that very often, on reaching the top of a staircase, you are out of breath, your heart is pounding, your legs are aching - and generally you could say that you are in a distressed state.

On other occasions, when your body is well balanced and nicely co-ordinated, you move up the stairs without getting into that distressed state. Why is this? Well, obviously, on those occasions you are maintaining the working integrity of yourself while climbing the stairs. This means

that all the neuromuscular connections, the muscles themselves and all the joints involved are working in harmony, no one part overworking, no one part underworking. Above all your breathing, which has, no doubt, become fuller as a result of this (or any other) activity, can remain in rhythm: there is no need for you to hold your breath, for it to become erratic or otherwise disturbed in such a way that the harmony of the movement is lost.

'Effortless action' is a term sometimes used to refer to a way of moving in harmony with the breath. It is found in a number of activities; among the first that come to mind is Tai Chi Ch'uan. Tai Chi, when practised over a number of years, becomes a graceful, flowing, harmonious way of moving, sometimes described as a 'moving meditation'. A mind totally absorbed in the movement to a point of stillness allows 'Chi' energy to 'do' the movement. The individual's awareness expands into 'non-doing' action.

That is the perfect action: flowing through you, with all levels of yourself - physical, mental, emotional, psychological and spiritual - in total harmony.

## Conscious awareness

The first thing we need to do

is to develop awareness of our 'misuse' of ourselves (that is, of where we are going wrong when we move). This is not always as easy as it might seem, because we are all caught up in the problem of unreliable sensory appreciation. This means that our senses may not register accurately how we are using ourselves when we are engaged in habitual, automatically programmed movement patterns.

Having become aware of our misuse, we next need to learn to inhibit those responses that interfere with the working integrity of ourelves, and substitute more appropriate ones. Inhibition in this sense does not mean suppressing movement or tightening muscles in any way, trying not to 'do' by effort. On the contrary, it means refusing to initiate the old response by intervening with the mind first - saying 'no' to the old, automatically programmed movement.

We then find that the space between the stimulus to move and our response allows us the time to reorganise our actions, and to gain understanding of a new and more appropriate way of using ourselves. The best method yet developed to accomplish this is, I believe, the one developed by F. M. Alexander.*

## Natural body poise

'A nice balance of superim-posed, irregularly shaped segments of bone, held together by strong ligaments and muscles, and motivated by muscles, which are controlled by the nervous system, is good body poise' - so says William Truslow in his book *Body Poise*. Unfortunately this is very rarely seen in modern human beings. Instead, uneven and asymmetrical development is the norm.

The co-ordination movements presented in the following pages are intended to go some way towards redressing this imbalance. An opportunity to explore symmetrical development and neuromuscular re-education is offered here. Do give it a try - it could be a decisive turning point in your life

*F. M. Alexander (1869-1955), developed a technique for expanding conciousness to take in inhibition as well as excitation, thus producing a better integration of the reflex and voluntary elements in the response pattern.
He went on to apply the principles he learnt in teaching others, influencing many well known people. The Aexander Technique is now widely used by many people who suffer from stress and the strain of modern living, and those having a pathological condition of one sort or another.*

# Joints and their Range of Movement (ROM)

The joints that are used most throughout this book are shown on these two pages. Knowing the location of joints is most important. Knowing where to bend from, and what a particular joint's range of movement is, will definitely be useful for you. Study the joint positions carefully. Some people find that it helps to think of yourself as a skeleton when you move. Try it!

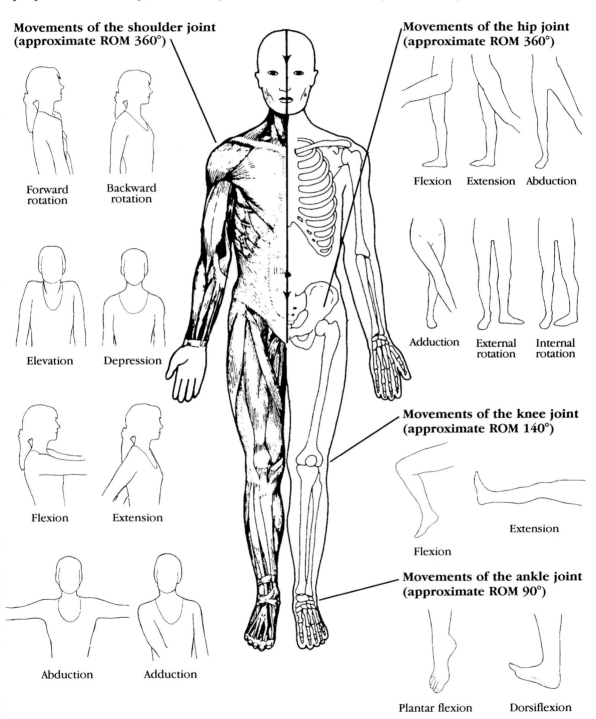

**Movements of the shoulder joint (approximate ROM 360°)**

Forward rotation    Backward rotation

Elevation    Depression

Flexion    Extension

Abduction    Adduction

**Movements of the hip joint (approximate ROM 360°)**

Flexion    Extension    Abduction

Adduction    External rotation    Internal rotation

**Movements of the knee joint (approximate ROM 140°)**

Flexion    Extension

**Movements of the ankle joint (approximate ROM 90°)**

Plantar flexion    Dorsiflexion

# The vertebral column

## The coordination of muscle action

The muscle which carries out a voluntary movement is called the 'agonist' or prime mover. The muscle which opposes the movement (although it actually facilitates it) is called the 'antagonist'. Muscles which help to stabilise joints and the body as a whole to allow other movements to take place are called 'synergists'.

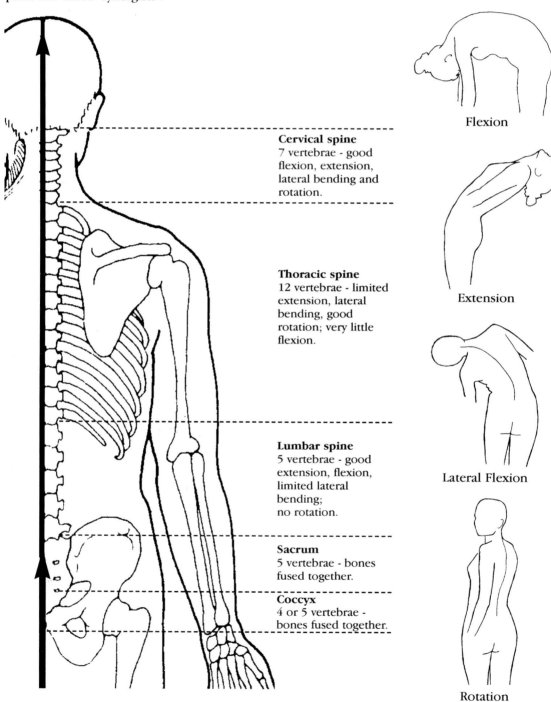

**Cervical spine**
7 vertebrae - good flexion, extension, lateral bending and rotation.

**Thoracic spine**
12 vertebrae - limited extension, lateral bending, good rotation; very little flexion.

**Lumbar spine**
5 vertebrae - good extension, flexion, limited lateral bending; no rotation.

**Sacrum**
5 vertebrae - bones fused together.

**Coccyx**
4 or 5 vertebrae - bones fused together.

Flexion

Extension

Lateral Flexion

Rotation

# Working with this book

The Golden Rule that applies to all the movements in this book is: if in any doubt, always check with your medical adviser before practising. Be aware of your own limitations, and keep within them.

Take time to rest for a few minutes before you embark on a series of procedures. Notice your breathing becoming more relaxed, and observe its natural rhythm. Your awareness of this natural rhythm is very important, because it will govern the speed of movement of your arms and legs.

Do remember that these movements are not 'exercises' that can be done without thinking. On the contrary, their purpose is to make you more aware of how you are moving, and the 'observations' that accompany the description of every procedure are intended to help you in this respect. Relax after you have completed a given procedure, too, and take the time to review it in your mind.

As you progress through the different movement patterns you should discover the answers to some or all of the following questions:

- where do I feel most discomfort and/or effort?

- which side of me moves more easily?

- what range of movement do I have on each side, compared with the other?

- how can I improve the quality of what I am doing?

You should also experience how movement becomes easier when body and mind are working harmoniously together.

Because it is so difficult for **us to** be able to feel accurately what we are doing when we move, a full-length mirror is worth its weight in gold for the extra visual feedback that it offers. Using one can greatly assist your growing awareness and understanding of how you are moving. Obviously the lying down positions do not lend themselves to observation by means of a mirror; in this case working with a friend, taking it in turns to observe and monitor each other's movements, can be equally advantageous.

Visualising the movements, repeating them several times in your mind before attempting them, helps to establish the requisite neuro-muscular connections. When you actually carry out the movements they will seem - and probably be - easier.

To assist you in following the written details of each procedure, the description of that part of it which is to be completed as you breathe out is printed in italics.

# Notes on the movement patterns

## Lying down in the supine position (10 procedures)

We start with lying down because it is the safest position in which to begin the movement patterns: the body is more relaxed, and there is no risk of falling over!

To encourage greater awareness, make sure you are lying in a straight line: that is, with your head, neck and trunk in alignment and your legs and feet equidistant from the mid-line of your body. You will then notice more readily any imbalances in arm or leg movements.

The lying-down procedures become progressively more difficult, thereby challenging your ability to maintain the integrity of your breathing and its natural rhythm. The two advanced lying-down co-ordination movements are included as a challenge to the more fit and able student. They should not be attempted by anyone with a pathological condition that would be a contra-indication.

## Standing movements (7 procedures)

The standing movements using the arms (5 procedures) allow action in a variety of directions through the full range of movement of the shoulder joint. The standing movements using the legs (two procedures) bring the hip joints into action.

## Walking in rhythm

This is a reminder of how important, and yet how underrated, walking is in keeping fit. I trust that all readers of this book will take the advice offered in the relevant pages and experience the joy and exhilaration of a good walk!

## Sitting down movements, using the arms (2 procedures)

The sitting-down movements using the arms are similar to the standing ones. They will be useful for anyone who finds difficulty in standing.

## Lying down in semi-supine (9 procedures)

This section offers the opportunity to gain maximum length through the spine with minimum effort while moving. This can be achieved by supporting your head on a firm block of foam rubber or a pile of books, the height of which is individually determined. It is useful to have a friend help you judge this: if it is too low, your neck will arch and no lengthening will occur in the cervical region of your spine. As a rule of thumb, it is better to have too much height than too little.

## Simple cross-patterning

Cross-patterning to help integrate the brain's two hemispheres is now widely recognised as a way of enhancing your learning ability - so a little time spent on this aspect of movement may well be rewarded.

## Background Music

Music is recommended to create an enjoyable climate which is conducive to learning. Choice of music is, of course, a matter of personal preference, but as long as it promotes a holistic balance between seeing, hearing and feeling, the three main ways of learning, it would be beneficial. You should feel free to add background music, though I would recommend you play it at a low volume for the best effect.

## Joint location

Shoulders (ball and socket)

## Approximate ROM

Shoulders 180°

## Starting position

Lying down with head, neck and trunk in a straight line. Feet and legs slightly apart, feet dropping outwards. Arms slightly away from the body, palms down. Body relaxed. Breathing relaxed. Note breathing rhythm, and use it to time the movement.

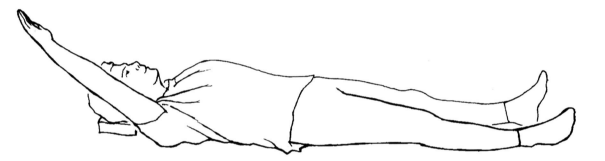

## The movement

As you breathe in, your right arm travels backwards to touch the floor behind your head exactly as your lungs are full.

*As you breathe out, your right arm travels forwards, coming back alongside your body exactly as your lungs are empty.*

Repeat this movement with the other arm. Then continue, using each arm alternately, for several minutes.

## Observations

● Make sure the movement of your arm synchronises exactly with your breath, and maintain the breathing rhythm throughout the sequence.

● Check that your arm is halfway through its movement when your lungs are half full, or half empty, of air.

● Refine your observation: is your arm following exactly the movement of your breath, from start to finish? Is your arm a quarter of the way through the movement when your lungs are a quarter full? An eighth of the way ... and so on?

# Lying-down movements (2)

## Joint location

Shoulders (ball and socket)

## Approximate ROM

Shoulders 180°

## Starting position

Lying down with head, neck and trunk in a straight line. Arms alongside your body, palms down. Breathing relaxed; note breathing rhythm.

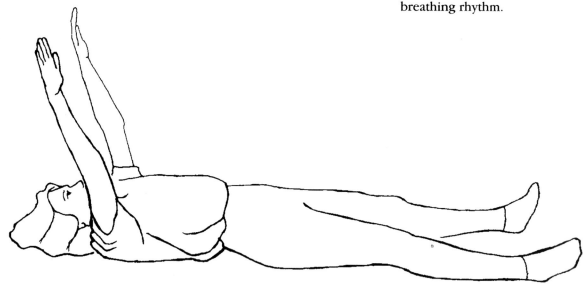

## The movement

As you breathe in, both arms travel backwards over your head to touch the floor behind it exactly when your lungs are full.

*As you breathe out, both arms travel forwards, coming back to the floor exactly as your lungs empty.*

## Observations

● Notice, once you have moved your arms a few times: is one hand touching the floor before the other? If so, adjust your arms so that the backs of your hands touch the floor behind your head together, and come back to rest alongside your body together. This is not so easy to do at first, but with a little practice you will improve.

● Is the movement of your arms synchronised with your breath?

● Does one arm move more freely? We all have an easier or freer side - no one is perfectly symmetrical.

## Joint location

Shoulders (ball and socket)

## Approximate ROM

Shoulders 180°

## Starting position

Lying down with head, neck and trunk in a straight line. Legs slightly apart, feet dropping outwards. Arms alongside your body, palms down. Breathing relaxed.

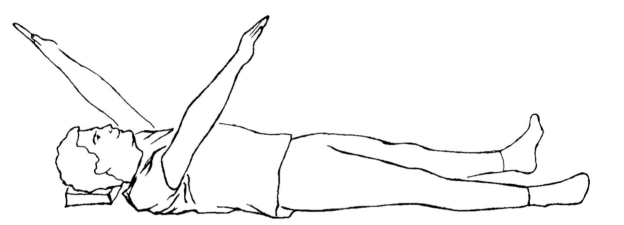

## The movement

As you breathe in, your left arm travels back over your head to touch the floor just as your lungs are full.

*As you breathe out, your left arm travels forwards, and your right arm backwards. Your left hand touches the floor alongside your body, and the back of your right hand touches the floor behind your head, just as your lungs ar empty.*

Continue moving your arms alternately forwards and back, exactly synchronised with your breathing.

## Observations

- After several movements, notice if one hand touches the floor before the other one? If so, make whatever adjustment is necessary to bring them down together. This may not be easy at first, but with 100% awareness of what you are doing you will find your co-ordination improving.

## Starting position

Lying down with head, neck and trunk in a straight line.
Arms alongside your body, palms down.
Breathing relaxed.
Notice the position of your lower back in relation to the floor.

## Joint location

Hips (ball and socket)

## Approximate ROM

Hips 90°

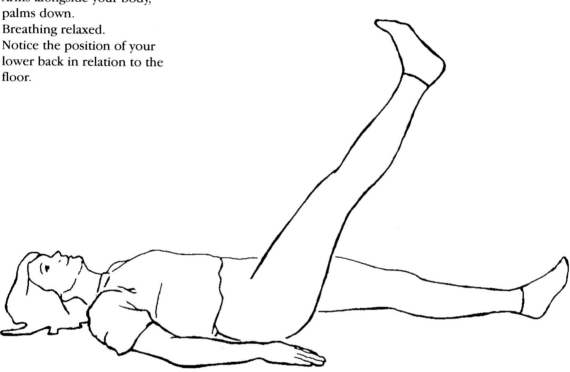

## The movement

As you breathe in, raise your left leg to its highest point.

*As you breathe out, lower your leg back to the floor.*

Repeat the movement, with your left leg this time.

Repeat movements with alternate legs an even number of times (say ten), and then rest, breathing easily.

## Observations

- As legs are heavier than arms, leg movements require more enegy.

- Make sure your breathing stays constant, without holding or interfering with it in any way.

- See that your leg moves in time with your breathing rhythm, so that it reaches its highest point exactly as your lungs are full, and your heel touches the floor exactly as they are empty.

- Check that your lower back stays easily in contact with the floor. If your lower back lifts up, discontinue the movement.

- You may find it helpful, if you have tight 'hamstrings' (the muscles that run down the back of your thighs), to soften the knee joint as you lift your leg, allowing it to bend slightly. This reduces the stretch on the hamstrings.

# Lying-down movements (5)

## Starting position

Lying down with head, neck and trunk in a straight line. Arms by your sides, palms down.
Breathing relaxed.

## Joint location

Shoulders (ball and socket)
Hips (ball and socket)

## Approximate ROM

Shoulders 180ø
Hips 90°

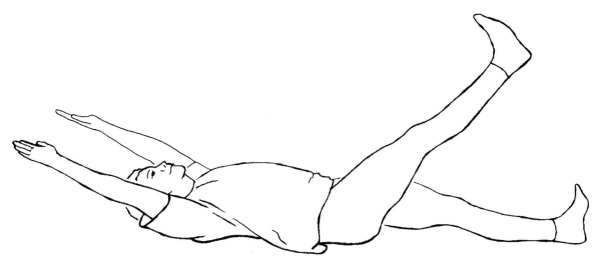

## The movement

As you breathe in, both arms travel backwards overhead, and you raise your right leg. As your lungs are filled, the backs of your hands touch the floor and your leg reaches its highest point.

*As you breathe out, both arms travel forwards and you lower your right leg. Your heel and both hands touch the floor together.*

Repeat the movement, using alternate legs each time, ten times in all.

## Observations

● As arms and leg travel at different speeds, 100% awareness is required.

● The leg, being heavier than the arms, needs more energy to move it. Be careful that your breathing rhythm is undisturbed.

● For the first time you are moving arms and leg together, so you have three things to focus on: your breathing, first and foremost; the movement of your arms, and the movement of your leg (which is slower than that of your arms).

● Most people, doing this for the first time, may have some difficulty with it. Be easy on yourself, and with practice you will find your co-ordination improving noticeably.

## Joint location

Shoulders (ball and socket)
Hips (ball and socket)

## Approximate ROM

Shoulders 180°
Hips 90°

## Starting position

Lying down, with head, neck and trunk in a straight line.
Arms by your sides, palms down.
Breathing relaxed.
Note the position of your lower back in relation to the floor.

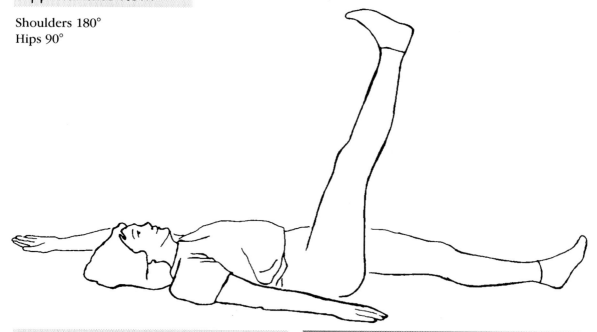

## The movement

As you breathe in, your right arm and left leg travel up and back. Your leg reaches its highest point as the back of your right hand touches the floor behind your head.

*As you breathe out, your right arm and leg travel forwards. Your hand comes to rest alongside your body as the heel of your left foot touches the floor.*

Repeat this movement, using your left arm and right leg.

Repeat both movements five more times, then rest. Review the movement in your mind. How well did you synchronise the movement with your breathing rhythm?

## Observations

- Using an opposite arm and leg can be a great deal easier than some of the other movements, because the body tends to be better balanced in cross-patterning.

- Obviously, the arm and leg move at different speeds, so you need to be very aware of how you are moving.

- From these procedures you develop the ability to focus on several things at once. It's a little like learning to drive a car: you think at first that no one could possibly attend to everything at once - changing gear, using the pedals, looking in the rear-view mirror, watching out for other traffic, steering... 'Impossible!' you say. Then, later on, you can drive and even listen to the radio, all at the same time!

## Joint location

Shoulders (ball and socket)
Hips (ball and socket)

## Approximate ROM

Shoulders 180°
Hips 90°

## Starting position

Lying down, with head, neck and trunk in a straight line.
Arms by your sides, palms down.
Breathing relaxed.
Note the position of your lower back
in relation to the floor.

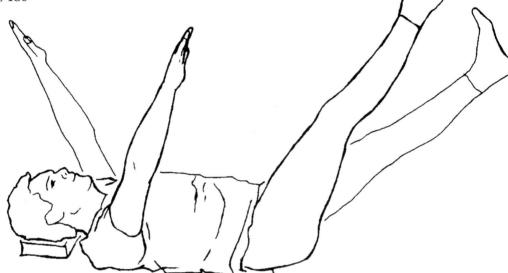

## The movement

As you breathe in, your right arm travels back
and you lift your left leg. The back of your
hand touches the floor behind your head as
your leg reaches its highest point.

*As you breathe out, your right arm and left leg
travel forwards, and at the same time you lift
your left arm and right leg. Opposite arms and
legs pass each other at the halfway point.*

Repeat the movement up to five times, then
rest for a few moments. How well did you do?

## Observations

● This is quite a demanding movement to master. It
requires 100% awareness. The tendency to hold the
breath is strong, but if you continue to focus on maintaining your breathing rhythm, the movement will
start to become easier.

● Make sure that your lower back stays in contact with
the floor, or in the same relation to it as when you
began. If you find your lower back lifting up, or
experience any discomfort, stop.

● These movements are designed not to develop
strength, stamina or endurance, but to refine your co-
ordination skills. However, we do need to 'play with
our limits' now and again. Never be afraid to do this,
once you have 'warmed up' and your co-ordination
has begun to improve.

## Joint location

Shoulders (ball and socket)
Hips (ball and socket)
Knees (hinge)

## Approximate ROM

Shoulders 180°
Hips 90°
Knees 120°

## Starting position

Lying down with head, neck and trunk in a straight line. Arms by your sides, palms down.
Breathing relaxed.

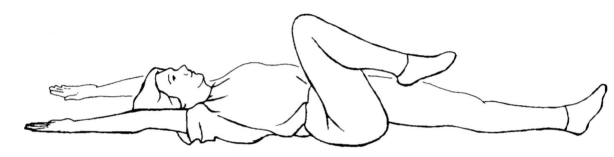

## The movement

As you breathe in, both arms travel back and your right knee moves towards your chest. At the moment your lungs are full, the backs of both hands touch the floor behind your head and your right knee arrives as close as it will come to your chest.

*As you breathe out, both arms travel forward and your right leg straightens up. At the moment your lungs are empty, both hands arrive back alongside your body and your right leg finally becomes straight.*

On the next in-breath, your arms travel back once more and your right knee comes back down towards your chest. As your lungs become full, the backs of both hands touch the floor behind your head and your knee arrives as close as it will come to your chest.

*As you breathe out, your arms move forward and your right leg straightens towards the floor. As the out-breath is completed, your right heel touches the floor and your hands return to the floor alongside your body.*

Repeat this sequence, using your left leg, with both arms moving together as before. Do four rounds, and return to a position of rest. Review your movements in your mind, and consider how well you were able to co-ordinate yourself.

## Observations

● This is a co-ordination movement in four stages, and, as you can see, it builds on the movements that you have learned so far. We are developing more complex movements for you to test yourself with, and, as you become more aware of how you are moving, you will find yourself coping with them with increased confidence.

● If you find your lower back lifting up, or if you experience any discomfort, stop. Remember, these movements are designed not to develop strength, stamina or endurance, but to refine your co-ordination skills.

# Lying-down movements (9 - advanced)

## Joint location

Shoulders (ball and socket)
Hips (ball and socket)
Spine (gliding)

## Starting position

Lying semi-supine, with feet,
knees and hips in line.
Arms by your sides, palms
down.
Breathing relaxed.

## Approximate ROM

Shoulders 180°
Hips 90°
Spine 90°

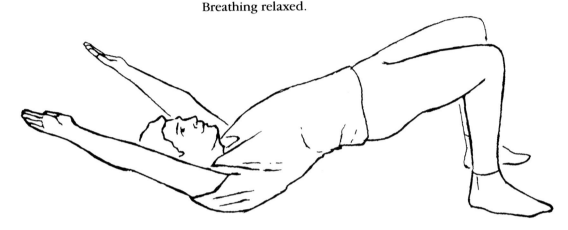

## The movement

As you breathe in, both arms travel back, your
hips lift up, and the backs of your hands touch
the floor behind your head as your spine arch-
es fully upwards.

*As you breathe out, both arms move forwards
while your hips and back continue arching
upwards. Both hands simultaneously touch the
floor alongside your body.*

As you breathe in, your arms travel back as
before, while your hips
and back continue arching upwards.

*As you breathe out, your arms move forwards
again, and you begin to lower your spine,
unrolling one vertebra at a time, from your
neck downwards, until, just as your lungs
become empty, your hips and hands simultaneously regain contact with the floor.*

## Observations

• Do not attempt this movement until you are familiar
with the previous procedures for developing co-ordination.

• This is an advanced movement, which asks you to
extend your spine. This will tend to limit or restrict
your breathing. Maintain rhythmic breathing, even
though it may be slightly shallow. This will allow your
arms to move in an easier, more effortless way.

• How high you raise your hips, and the degree of
extension of your spine, are not the important points
in this movement. People with a naturally loose spine
will be able to lift their hips quite high and still maintain good use of themselves - but do not try to com-
pete with them! Rather, it is ease and smoothness of
movement that you should be aiming for.

• Take time to analyse your movements before going on
to the next procedure, learning in the process to make
all the necessary adjustments to harmonise the move
ment with your breathing. Remember to maintain the
working integrity of yourself.

# Lying-down movements (10 - advanced)

## Joint location

Shoulders (ball and socket)
Hips (ball and socket)
Spine (gliding)

## Approximate ROM

Shoulders 180°
Hips 90°
Spine 90°

## Starting position

Lying semi-supine, with feet
and knees together.
Arms by your sides, palms
down.
Breathing relaxed.

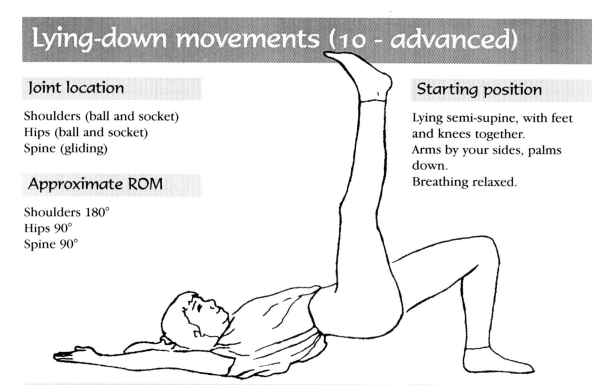

## The movement

As you breathe in, both arms travel back and your hips lift up. Just as your lungs fill, the backs of your hands touch the floor behind your head and your hips and spine are arched fully upwards.

*As you breathe out, your arms move forwards, while your hips and back remain arching upwards. As your lungs empty, your hands return to the floor alongside your body.*

As you breathe in, both arms travel back once more, and at the same time you begin to lift your right leg. Just as your lungs fill, the backs of your hands touch the floor behind your head and your leg is extended fully upwards.

*As you breathe out, your arms move forwards. Your hips and back remain arching upwards as you lower your right leg. As your lungs empty, your foot and both hands simultaneously touch the floor.*

As you breathe in, both arms travel back once more, and at the same time you begin to lift your left leg. Your hips and back continue arching upwards. Just as your lungs fill, the backs of your hands touch the floor behind your head, and your leg is extended fully upwards.

*As you breathe out, your arms move forwards. Your hips and back continue arching upwards as you lower your left leg. As your lungs empty, your foot and both hands simultaneously touch the floor.*

As you breathe in, both arms travel back. Your hips and spine remain arching upwards. As your lungs fill, the backs of your hands touch the floor behind your head.

*As you breathe out, your arms move forwards, and you begin to unroll your spine, one vertebrae at a time, from the neck downwards. As your lungs empty, your hips and hands touch the floor simultaneously.*

Rest, and then repeat the sequence.

## Observations

● This is another advanced movement, requiring great awareness and attention to detail.

● Let your neck be soft, and direct your head away from the top of your spine, thus maintaining optimum length in your spine throughout the movement.

● When you lift your leg with your body arched, the tendency to hold your breath will be strong - but do resist it! Endeavour to maintain even, rhythmic breathing, although it may be shallow and somewhat restricted. This is because your diaphragm is being stretched, and your ribs are held in a tight, more fixed position.

● For most people, this is the most demanding synchronised movement in The Movement Book. Therefore, if you do find your breathing rhythm disturbed, stop, return to a position of rest, and recover relaxed breathing. You will gain more proficiency and confidence if you go back to the simpler movements in the book and then try this one again later on.

## Joint location

Shoulders (ball and socket)

## Approximate ROM

Shoulders 360°

## Starting position

Standing, with feet hips' width apart.
Arms hanging loosely by your sides.
Breathing relaxed.

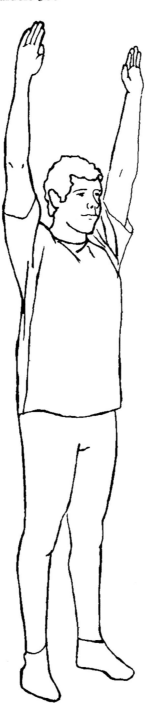

## The movement

As you breathe in, both arms move forwards and up, from the 6 o'clock position to the 12 o'clock position.

*As you breathe out, both arms travel back and down, from 12 o'clock to 6 o'clock.*

Repeat this circling movement ten times, then rest, shake your arms and ease out your shoulders.

## Observations

- Aim for a smooth, easy, rhythmical rotation of your arms, both moving together all the way round (not one in front of the other).

- Notice how freely each arm moves. Which is your looser side?

- Let your neck be free, and think of the head moving forward and up from the top joint of your neck, encouraging the spine to lengthen.

## Joint location

Shoulders (ball and socket)

## Approximate ROM

Shoulders 360°

## Starting position

Standing, with feet approximately hips' width apart.
Arms hanging loosely by your sides.
Breathing relaxed.

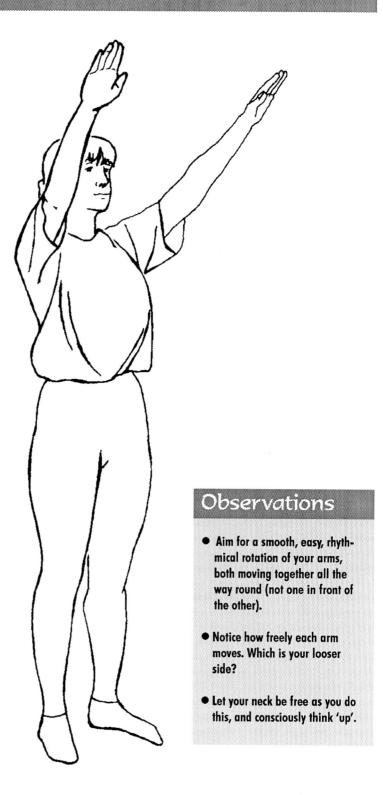

## The movement

As you breathe in, both arms move back and up, from the 6 o'clock position to the 12 o'clock position. Lungs filled.

*As you breathe out, both arms travel forwards and down, from 12 o'clock to 6 o'clock. Lungs empty.*

Repeat this circling movement ten times, then rest, and shake your arms loosely. How well did you harmonise the movement of your arms with your breathing?

## Observations

- Aim for a smooth, easy, rhythmical rotation of your arms, both moving together all the way round (not one in front of the other).

- Notice how freely each arm moves. Which is your looser side?

- Let your neck be free as you do this, and consciously think 'up'.

## Joint location

Shoulders (ball and socket)

## Approximate ROM

Shoulders 360°

## Starting position

Standing, with feet hips' width apart.
Head freely balanced on top of spine.
Right arm up, left arm down.
Breathing relaxed.

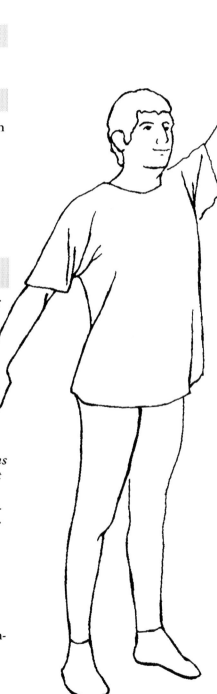

## The movement

As you breathe in, rotate your arms, right arm moving forward from 12 o'clock to 6 o'clock, left arm moving backwards from 6 o'clock to 12 o'clock. As your lungs are full, your left hand reaches its highest position.

*As you breathe out, your arms continue to rotate, your right arm moving backwards and up, your left arm moving forwards and down. When your lungs are empty, your left hand reaches its lowest position.*

Hands continue circling in opposition, at an angle of 180ø to one another, throughout the movement.

## Observations

- This movement is not quite as easy as it seems. To keep the arms in direct opposition to one another requires 100% awareness of what you are doing.

- Your arms circle slowly, keeping time with your breathing rhythm.

- When one hand is at the top, the other is at the bottom. When one hand is in front of you, the other is behind you.

- Allow the breath to move the arms. Focus on the breathing and you will notice the arms begin to move more freely.

## Joint location

Shoulders (ball and socket)

## Approximate ROM

Shoulders 360°

## Starting position

Standing, with feet hips' width apart.
Right arm straight up close to your ear, left arm by your side.
Breathing relaxed.

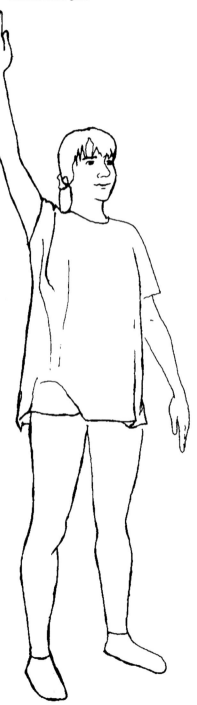

## The movement

As you breathe in, rotate both arms in a backwards direction, your right arm moving back and downward from the 12 o'clock to the 6 o'clock position, and your left arm moving forward and upward from the 6 o'clock to the 12 o'clock position.

*As you breathe out, your arms continue rotating backwards, your right arm moving from 6 o'clock to 12 o'clock, and your left arm moving from 12 o'clock to 6 o'clock.*

Repeat this movement ten times.

## Observations

● Your arms stay at an angle of 180° throughout the rotations, and move exactly in time with your breathing.

● Notice, do you get out of breath? If so, slow down.

● Always match the movement to your breathing, thereby maintaining the working integrity of yourself.

## Joint location

Shoulders (ball and socket)

## Starting position

Standing, with feet hips' width apart.
Arms hanging loosely by your sides.
Breathing relaxed.

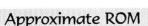

## Approximate ROM

Shoulders 360°

## The movement

As you breathe in, both arms travel outwards and upwards. Your hands reach their highest point as your lungs become full.

*As you breathe out, your arms continue to travel round and down, in front of your body, the left arm in front of the right. Your hands reach their lowest point as your lungs become empty.*

Continue circling your arms, your right and left arm alternately being to the front as they pass in front of your body.

After ten revolutions, to keep you thinking during this movement, reverse the direction of your arms so that they are circling outwards.

## Observations

● When you stop, remember to review your progress. What do you need to do to improve co-ordination?

● Check that the movement is as smooth as possible, with the rhythm of your breath governing the action the whole time.

● Aim to let your arms move effortlessly.

## Joint location

Hips (ball and socket)

## Approximate ROM

Hips 90°

## Starting position

Standing, with feet together.
Hands on hips.
Breathing relaxed.

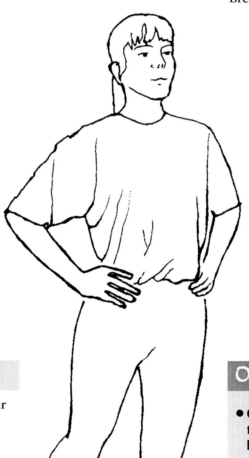

## The movement

As you breathe in, bend your left knee, lift your heel and foot off the floor and swing your leg forwards.

*As you breathe out, swing your left leg back, the same distance behind you as you did in front.*

Continue this movement, without strain, for ten breaths.

Rest, then repeat the sequence with the other leg.

## Observations

- Check that the your leg swings the same distance forwards and backwards.

- Check that your breathing rhythm is governing the movement of your leg.

- Balance with the minimum of effort, release tension from your neck, have your head poised directly above the support leg, keeping optimum length in your spine. Pelvis to be stabilised and kept in balance throughout the movement.

## Joint location

Hips (ball and socket)

## Approximate ROM

Hips 90°

## Starting position

Standing, with feet together.
Hands on hips.
Breathing relaxed.

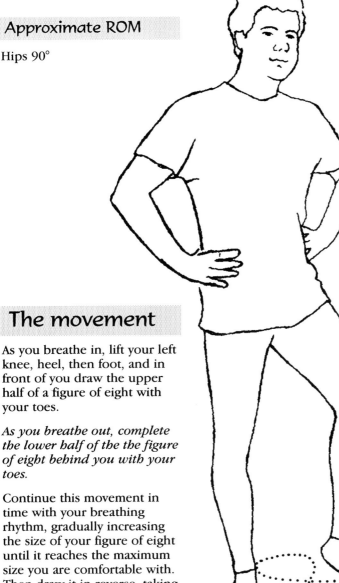

## The movement

As you breathe in, lift your left knee, heel, then foot, and in front of you draw the upper half of a figure of eight with your toes.

*As you breathe out, complete the lower half of the the figure of eight behind you with your toes.*

Continue this movement in time with your breathing rhythm, gradually increasing the size of your figure of eight until it reaches the maximum size you are comfortable with. Then draw it in reverse, taking your foot round in the opposite direction. Gradually reduce your figure of eight to the size you started with, then stop.

Repeat this sequence with your right foot.

## Observations

- Focus on synchronising the movement of your leg with the rhythm of your breathing.

- Balance with minimum effort, head, neck and trunk in line, use your hands to stabilise your pelvis and keep it in balance throughout the movement.

# Walking in rhythm

## Harmony and rhythm in everyday movement

Rhythm and good movement go together. They produce a harmony which shows in any action. There are many possible examples of this partnership - think of a rowing crew, a dance troupe, or marching soldiers. It is the same for individuals: when you move or work in rhythm, effort is reduced and your task is much easier. This is visible to an observer - and you can feel it yourself. It looks easier because it is easier!

Take walking, for example. When you are walking in rhythm you experience a much greater sense of freedom, with much less effort and a feeling of lightness in every step. So why not learn to walk with rhythm and harmony?

## Have you any imbalances?

To begin with, we need to look for any imbalances. Use a full-length mirror, or get a friend to help by watching you as you do the following movements.

First, stand with your feet together. Then lift your right leg, with your knee bent and your thigh parallel to the floor. Do your hips remain level as you do this? Repeat the movement with your left leg. Again, notice any tendency for your hips to tilt. Do you have balanced hips? You should be able to lift one leg without your hips tilting sideways! *(Fig. 1)*

Now let's view the same movement from the side.

*Fig. 1*

Remember that, if possible, you should lift your thighs into a position parallel with the floor. Again, notice any tendency for your hips to tilt, perhaps backwards or forwards this time? *(Fig.2)*

## We need to maintain balanced hips when we move

Any imbalance in these movements will be accentuated in walking, and if you were to take up jogging or running they would be even more pronounced, maybe even to the point of causing discomfort or pain which might eventually affect your ankle-, knee- or hip-joints, or your lower back. So you can begin to appreciate the need for your hips to be in balance as you walk.

Muscle groups, as well as joints involved in a particular movement, may be subject to inappropriate stress and strain - and so may other muscle groups not directly involved in that movement. The body works not in isolated parts but as an integrated whole, and what affects one part will eventually affect the rest.

Consider our use of ourselves in general, and you begin to see how important it is in avoiding 'wear and tear' for us to be well co-ordinated in our movements.

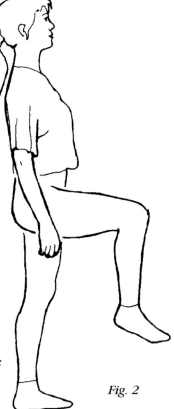

*Fig. 2*

## We need flexibility in our hips

Flexibility of the hip-joint involves the ability to turn your hips without turning your shoulders - or to turn your shoulders without turning your hips.

Try sitting in a chair and turning your upper body one way or the other, without moving your hips.

Or stand, facing a mirror, and twist your hips first one way and then the other, without moving your shoulders. This may not seem so easy at first, but with a litle practice you will soon get the feel of it.

Flexibility in the area of the low back and hips is vital for acquiring a good hip stride when you walk.

## Walking

Let us now take a closer look at the way you have been walking, to see if any noticeable improvement is possible.

Start, as always, with the working integrity of yourself. Your breathing is the key to this, so tune in to the rhythm of your breathing, and then be aware that in normal walking you do not need to disturb it.

*Fig. 3*

Begin by marking time on the spot, raising your knees but keeping your toes on the floor, and swinging your arms backwards and forwards. Your right arm swings forward as you raise your left knee, and your left arm swings forward as you raise your right knee. *(Fig 3)*

Now observe whether your right arm swings the same distance as your left. If not, make whatever adjustment is necessary to let both arms be the same in the length of their swing, forwards and backwards. *(Fig. 4)*

*Fig. 4*

If, at any stage while doing these movements, you feel fatigued or your attention wanders, stop. Have a rest, and begin again when you are ready.

Next, mark time as you lift each foot in turn fully off the floor, while both arms swing an equal distance, forwards and backwards. Use a mirror, or ask your friend to observe your movements to help you make any necessary adjustments.

Keep the movement going, and close your eyes. This gives you the opportunity to explore proprioceptive feeling - that is, your inner body-awareness, or sixth sense. By doing this many people will gain a fuller awareness of how they are moving.

## On to walking itself

As you stride away, notice the following points:

- easy, rhythmic movements producing effortless action, in which your whole body is involved

- strong but effortless hip stride. Walk 'off' your legs, not 'on' them, and think 'up' along the length of your spine

- let your stride be balanced, stepping the same distance forward with each leg - you could use the lines between paving stones to guide you

- let your arms move in a balanced way, equal in the length of their swing, for wards and backwards

- let your head be poised freely on the top of your spine, which lengthens upwards, with your hips balanced below

- let your feet be parallel to each other, toes pointing forwards

- let your breathing be relaxed and rhythmical

- follow the movement with your mind.

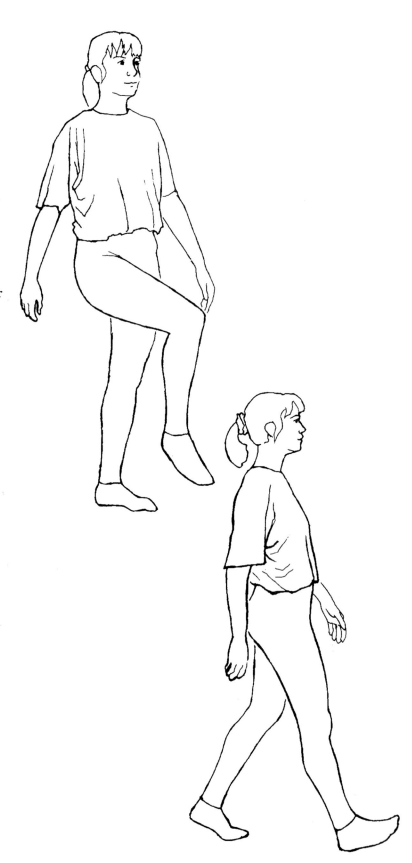

## Joint location

Shoulders (ball and socket)

## Approximate ROM

Shoulders 360°

## Starting position

Sitting comfortably.
Arms hanging loosely along-side your body.
Breathing relaxed.

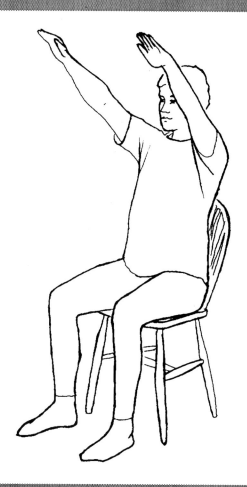

## The movement

As you breathe in, both arms travel back and up from the 6 o'clock to the 12 o'clock position, reaching 12 o'clock as your lungs are filled.

*As you breathe out, both arms continue to travel forwards from 12 o'clock to 6 o'clock, reaching 6 o'clock as your lungs empty.*

Repeat ten times, then relax, give your arms a thorough shake, and review the movements in your mind.

## Observations

● Arm-circling in harmony with the breath while sitting is similar to the movement which you did while standing. However, some people find it easier to focus clearly when sitting, so you may notice more, this time, about the way you move.

● Check that both arms move together as they rotate, and that one hand is not in advance of the other.

● Observe how the palms of your hands change direction, facing forwards as your arms rotate forwards, and inwards as your arms rotate backwards.

## Joint location

Shoulders (ball and socket)

## Approximate ROM

Shoulders 360°

## Starting position

Sitting comfortably.
Right arm hanging loosely by
your side.
Left arm up close to your ear.
Breathing relaxed.

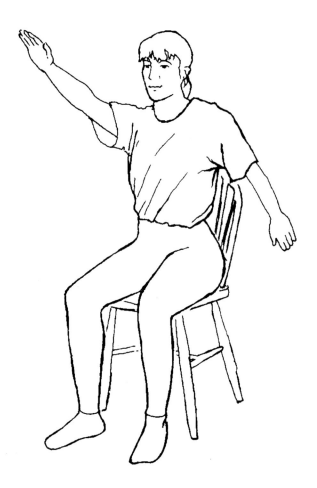

## The movement

As you breathe in, your right arm travels backwards and up from
the 6 o'clock to the 12 o'clock position, and your left arm moves
forwards and down from 12 o'clock to 6 o'clock. Both hands
reach their finishing position as your lungs are filled.

*As you breathe out, your right arm travels forwards and down
from 12 o'clock to 6 o'clock, and your left arm backwards and
up from 6 o'clock to 12 o'clock. Both hands reach their finishing position as your lungs are empty.*

Continue for ten revolutions of your arms, then rest. Consider
how well you synchronised the movement with your breathing.

## Observations

● Check, as you rotate your arms,
that they remain at an angle of
180°.

● Watch the integrity of yourself:
always let your breathing govern
the speed of the movement, and
always move within your own
capability.

# Semi-supine movements: arms (1)

## Joint location

Shoulders (ball and socket)

## Approximate ROM

Shoulders 180°

## Starting position

Lying down, with head, neck and trunk in a straight line.
Knees bent; feet hips' width apart.
Arms lying alongside your body, palms up.
Breathing relaxed.
Support head if required.

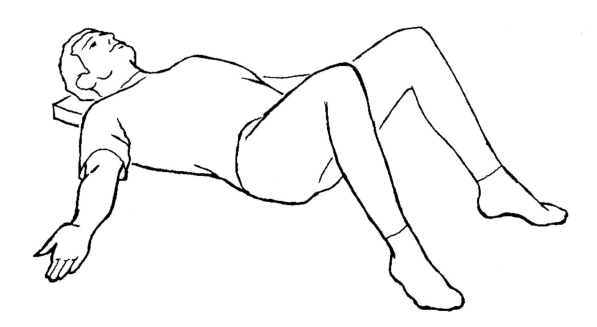

## The movement

As you breathe in, both arms circle round and back across the floor, arriving behind your head exactly as your lungs are filled.

*As you breathe out, both arms travel round and forwards, returning to rest alongside your body exactly as your lungs empty.*

Continue with this movement for ten breaths. Then rest, giving yourself time to reflect on how well you did.

## Observations

● Are your arms moving together, and arriving together?

● How accurate are you in keeping the movement in time with your breath?

## Joint location

Shoulders (ball and socket)

## Approximate ROM

Shoulders 180°

## Starting position

Lying down, with head, neck and trunk in a straight line.
Knees bent; feet hips' width apart.
Arms lying slightly away from the sides of your body, palms up.
Breathing relaxed. Support head if required.

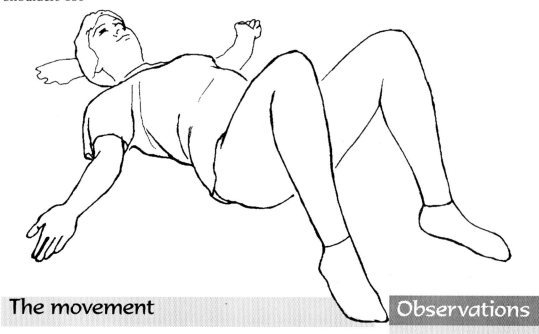

## The movement

As you breathe in, your right arm circles around the floor, coming to rest behind your head exactly as your lungs are filled.

*As you breathe out, your right arm travels forwards, while your left arm circles back behind your head. Exactly as your lungs empty, your right arm returns to rest alongside your body, and your left arm reaches its maximum extent.*

As you breathe in, your right arm travels back, and your left arm travels forwards. Exactly as your lungs are full, your right arm reaches its maximum extent, and your left arm comes to rest alongside your body.

*As you breathe out, your right arm travels forwards, and your left arm circles back behind your head. Exactly as your lungs empty, your right arm returns to rest alongside your body, and your left arm reaches its maximum extent.*

Continue with this movement of both arms for ten breaths, then rest, giving yourself time to reflect on how well you did.

## Observations

● Let your arms move together, at a constant angle of 180ø to one another.

● When your arms are at the halfway point, your lungs are half-empty, or half-full.

● Aim for a smooth, effortless action, with your movement regulated entirely by your breath.

## Joint location

Elbows (hinge)

## Approximate ROM

Elbows 90°

## Starting position

Lying down, with head, neck and trunk in a straight line. Knees bent; feet hips' width apart.
Arms lying slightly away from the sides of your body, palms up.
Breathing relaxed.
Support head if required.

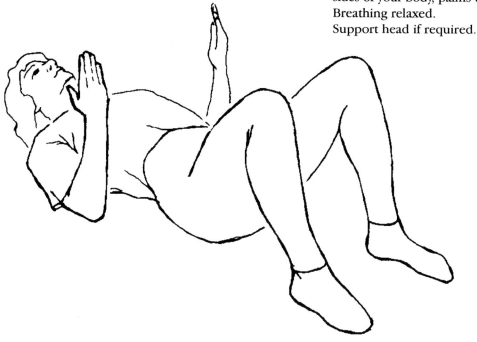

## The movement

As you breathe in, your hands and forearms move up into a vertical position, your elbows reaching an angle of 90ø exactly as your lungs are filled.

*As you breathe out, lower your hands and forearms back down, to reach the floor exactly as your lungs empty.*

Continue with this movement for ten breaths, then rest, and review how well you did.

## Observations

● As the arms are fairly light, focusing on yourself as you move is undemanding.

● Check that your arms are moving in unison. Both hands should reach the vertical position at the same time, and touch the floor at the same time.

● Check that you are staying in rhythm with your breath.

## Joint location

Elbows (hinge)

## Approximate ROM

Elbows 90°

## Starting position

Lying down, with head, neck and trunk in a straight line.
Knees bent; feet hips' width apart.
Arms lying slightly away from the sides of your body, palms up.
Breathing relaxed. Support head if required.

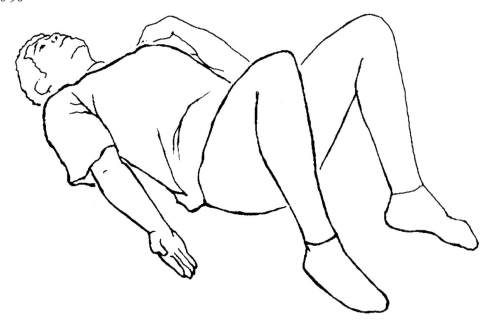

## The movement

As you breathe in, raise your left forearm so that your fingertips
touch your left shoulder exactly as your lungs are filled.

*As you breathe out, let your left forearm return towards the
floor, while you raise your right forearm. Exactly as your lungs
empty, the fingertips of your right hand touch your right shoulder, and your left hand touches the floor.*

As you breathe in, raise your left forearm, while your right forearm returns towards the floor. Exactly as your lungs are filled,
the fingertips of your left hand touch your left shoulder, and
your right hand touches the floor.

Continue with this alternating arm movement for ten breaths,
then return to a position of rest, with both arms alongside your
body and your breathing relaxed.

## Observations

- Moving your forearms in this way is quite simple, because they are light (in comparison, say, with your legs), making this movement an easy opportunity to synchronise the movement with your breathing.

- Do you begin to notice which muscle groups are involved in the movement? Where are you applying most effort? See if you can reduce the amount of effort, letting the movement be so smooth that it becomes almost effortless.

# Semi-supine movements: arms and legs (1)

## Joint location

Hips (ball and socket)
Elbows (hinge)

## Approximate ROM

Shoulders 30°
Elbows 90°

## Starting position

Lying down, with head, neck and trunk in a straight line. Head supported, if required.
Knees bent; feet hips' width apart.
Arms lying alongside your body, palms up.
Breathing relaxed.

## The movement

As you breathe in, you raise your left forearm and your right knee. Your forearm and thigh arrive at a vertical position as your lungs are filled.

*As you breathe out, lower your forearm and knee so that they regain their starting positions exactly as your lungs become empty.*

As you breathe in, you raise your right forearm and your left knee. Forearm and thigh arrive at a vertical position as your lungs are filled.

*As you breathe out, lower your forearm and knee so that they regain their starting position exactly as your lungs become empty.*

Continue moving alternate arms and legs in this way for ten breaths. Then return to a position of rest, and reflect on how well you did the movements.

## Observations

- This is a four-part sequence, which gives you a great opportunity to observe the range of movement on either side of your body.

- As your arm and leg are moving at different speeds, take care to keep the action in exact time with your breath.

## Joint location

Hips (ball and socket)
Elbows (hinge)

## Approximate ROM

Shoulders 30°
Elbows 90°

## Starting position

Lying down, with head, neck and trunk in a straight line. Head supported, if required.
Knees bent; feet hips' width apart.
Arms lying alongside your body, palms up.
Breathing relaxed.

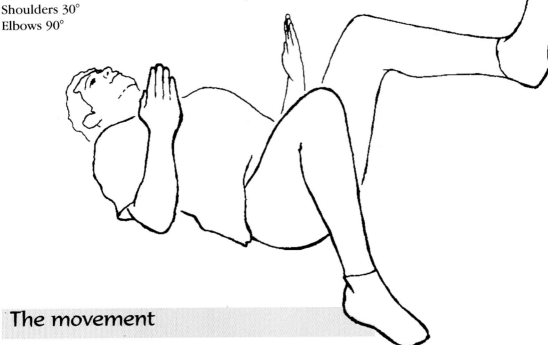

## The movement

As you breathe in, raise both forearms and your right knee. Your forearms and thigh arrive at a vertical position exactly as your lungs are filled.

*As you breathe out, lower your forearms and leg so that your hands and heel touch the floor exactly as your lungs become empty.*

As you breathe in, you raise both forearms and your left knee. Forearms and thigh arrive at a vertical position exactly as your lungs are filled.

*As you breathe out, lower your forearms and leg so that your hands and heel regain contact with the floor exactly as your lungs become empty.*

Continue moving your forearms and alternate legs in this way for ten breaths. Then return to a position of rest, and reflect on how well you did the movements.

## Observations

- Here again, we have a four-part sequence with arms and legs moving at different speeds. This demands an expanded awareness in order to carry out and keep track of what this movement requires.

# Semi-supine movements: arms and legs (3)

## Joint location

Hips (ball and socket)
Neck (gliding)

## Approximate ROM

Hips 90°
Neck 90°

## Starting position

Lying down, with head, neck and trunk in a straight line.
Knees bent; feet hips' width apart.
Arms lying alongside your body, palms up.
Breathing relaxed.
Head supported, as required.

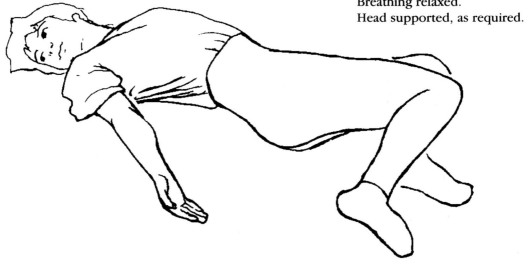

## The movement

*As you breathe out, both knees move to the right and your head rotates to the left. Knees and head reach their maximum degree of rotation exactly as your lungs are empty.*

As you breathe in, your knees and your head simultaneously travel back, reaching a central position exactly as your lungs are full.

*As you breathe out, both knees move to the left and your head rotates to the right. Knees and head reach their maximum degree of rotation exactly as your lungs are empty.*

As you breathe in, your knees and your head simultaneously travel back to reach a central position exactly as your lungs are full.

Continue this contra-rotation of your knees and head, both synchronised with the rhythm of your breathing, for ten breaths.

## Observations

- This is a cross-patterning action, so you should find it easy to perform.

- Aim for a smooth, rhythmical action, with head and knees moving freely.

- Reduce the amount of effort used until the movement becomes effortless.

- Remember to let your breathing determine the speed of movement at all times.

# Semi-supine movements: advanced (1)

## Joint location

Hips (ball and socket)
Elbows (hinge)
Neck (gliding)

## Approximate ROM

Hips  30°
Elbows 90°
Neck 90°

## Starting position

Lying, with head, neck and
trunk in a straight line.
Knees bent.
Arms lying alongside your
body, palms up.
Breathing relaxed.
Head supported, if required.

## The movement

*As you breathe out, both your forearms move up, both knees
travel to the right and your head to the left. As your lungs are
empty, your forearms reach the vertical position, your knees
reach maximum rotation to the right and your head maximum
rotation to the left.*

As you breathe in, you lower your forearms, and your knees and
head return towards the centre. Exactly as your lungs become
full, the backs of your hands touch the floor and your knees and
head regain the central position.

*As you breathe out, both your forearms move up, both knees
travel to the left and your head to the right. As your lungs are
empty, your forearms reach the vertical position, your knees
reach maximum rotation to the left and your head maximum
rotation to the right.*

As you breathe in, you lower your forearms, and your knees and
head return towards the centre. Exactly as your lungs become
full, the backs of your hands touch the floor and your knees and
head regain the central position.

Repeat this movement several times, then rest, and review it.

## Observations

● This is a complex movement that
really tests your co-ordination
skills!

● With your head, arms and legs
all moving at different speeds,
can you synchronise all the
movements with your breathing
rhythm?

● Can you refine the movement so
as to use the minimum of effort?

## Joint location

Hips (ball and socket)
Elbows (hinge)
Neck (gliding)

## Approximate ROM

Hips  30°
Elbows 90°
Neck 90°

## Starting position

Lying down, with head, neck and trunk in a straight line.
Knees bent. Head supported, if required.
Arms lying alongside your body, palms up.
Breathing relaxed.

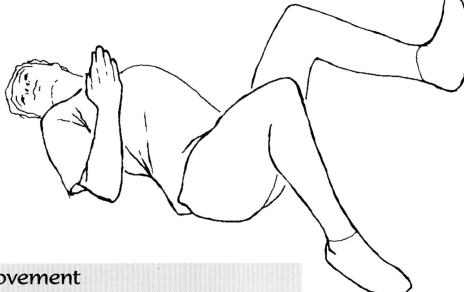

## The movement

As you breathe in, your left forearm and right knee move
upwards and your head rotates towards the left. As your lungs
are filled, your forearm and thigh reach the vertical position and
your head reaches its maximum degree of rotation.

*As you breathe out, your left forearm and right knee move
downwards and your head rotates towards the right. Exactly
as your lungs are empty, your foot and hand touch the floor
and your head returns to the central position.*

As you breathe in, your right forearm and left knee move
upwards and your head rotates towards the right. As your lungs
are filled, your forearm and thigh reach the vertical position and
your head reaches its maximum degre of rotation.

*As you breathe out, your right forearm and left knee move
downwards and your head rotates towards the left. Exactly as
your lungs are empty, your foot and hand touch the floor and
your head returns to the central position.*

Repeat this movement several times, then rest, and review it.

## Observations

● **This movement gives you a great
deal to think about! You will
need time to allow the neuromuscular pathways to become
established. Then you can begin
to refine the way you move.**

# Hands-and-knees position

### Joint location

Hips (ball and socket)
Shoulders (ball and socket)

### Approximate ROM

Hips 90°
Shoulders 90°

### Starting position

On all fours, supporting your-self from your hands and knees.
Back flat.
Arms and thighs vertical.
Breathing relaxed.

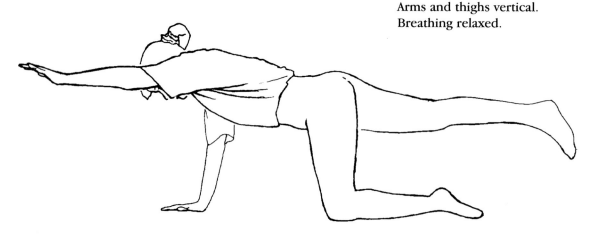

## The movement

As you breathe in, your left arm begins to move forwards and your right leg back, both reaching a horizontal position exactly as your lungs are filled.

*As you breathe out, let your arm and leg descend, your hand and knee touching the floor exactly as your lungs become empty.*

As you breathe in, your right arm begins to move forwards and your left leg back, both reaching a horizontal position exactly as your lungs are filled.

*As you breathe out, let your arm and leg descend, your hand and knee touching the floor exactly as your lungs become empty.*

Repeat the movement with alternate arms and legs for ten breaths, then rest.

## Observations

- Here is a cross-patterning move ment which also involves an element of balance.

- Because it uses opposite arms and legs, you should find this movement helps towards de-rotation of the trunk and a general realignment of the spine.

- Aim for smooth lifting of your limbs, synchronised with your breathing rhythm.

- Once your limbs are horizontal, direct your fingers and toes away from your body. Maintain a free neck and a flat back throughout.

# Overdoing

Most people, unlike animals when they move, use far more effort and energy than is required. This we call overdoing!

Here is an opportunity to find out whether you are using more muscular effort than you need to, by carrying out the following exercise.

Lie in the semi-supine position, your hands resting lightly on your abdomen with the fingers touching. A few books under your head will help release tension in your neck and encourage your spine to lengthen.

First, give yourself the order to extend your right leg forward. Then extend it, observing how you move it. Use this observational awareness checklist to help you:

● where did you feel most effort?

● which major muscle groups were involved in moving your leg?

● did other muscle groups, unrelated to the task of moving your leg, contract?

● did you notice anything happening in your other, stationary leg?

● did anything happen to your breathing?

● what happened to your neck muscles?

Now bring your leg back into the semi-supine position.

## Anticipating movement

Again, give yourself the instruction to extend your right leg - but this time, just as you are about to carry out the instruction and lift your foot off the floor, transfer the intention to move to your other leg!

Continue to play this game with yourself, forming the intention of lifting one leg, and at the last instant transferring the planned movement to the other leg. In this way you will discover how you anticipate the movement, and how much effort you are making with your muscles before the event.

## Undoing unnecessary effort

You will now be able to reduce the effort you habitually apply, by consciously learning to inhibit your old response to the stimulus to move. In this way you will re-educate the use of yourself in a manner more appropriate to the task.

For example, if you noticed how much effort you were applying to the task of lifting your leg, see if you can reduce it - not only in the muscles that move your leg, but also in those that are merely acting as stabilisers in your stationary leg.

You may have noticed your neck muscles tensing as you lifted and moved your leg. If so, focus on your neck muscles, letting them be soft and relaxed next time you move your leg, and observe the result: you should find your leg moving more freely and with much less effort.

# Simple cross-patterning

Bilateral movement, or cross-patterning, plays an important part in integrating the two hemispheres of the brain. The left hemisphere controls movement on the right side of the body, and the right hemisphere controls movement on the left side.

The left hemisphere also relates to language, rational and sequential thought, logical reasoning and objective analysis. The right hemisphere is concerned with how things relate to one another, and with shapes, patterns and images; it also governs our intuitive sense.

## The holistic approach

People learn more quickly and easily when the two hemispheres are working together, rather than one being dominant. Activating both sides of the body helps to integrate the two hemispheres.

This can induce a meditative state of mind in which total balance equals 'no thought' and produces instead 'expanded awareness'. In this state body and mind are in total harmony. Some athletes experience it, especially in rhythmical activities like cycling or running; a number of runners have described it as 'runner's high'. Moving in this state is experienced as truly 'effortless action'.

## Crawling

In a kneeling position on all fours, check first that your back is flat and straight. This is not easy to do, as you cannot see your back and your feelings are not always reliable. A friend could help you by giving feedback and assisting you in making any necessary adjustments.

Always direct your head forwards, letting it lead the movement.

### 1/4 time

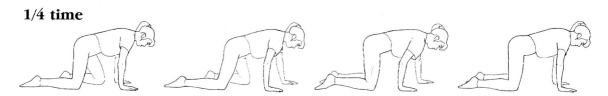

Direct your head forwards as you slide your left knee forwards. Then your left hand moves forwards; then your right knee, followed by your right hand. Continue this sequence: knee, hand, knee, hand.

Aim for a smooth, rhythmical, flowing forward movement. Let your breathing be relaxed and easy.

### 1/2 time

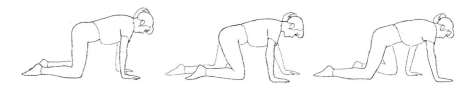

Start from a kneeling position, as for 1/4 time crawling. This follows on from 1/4, but it allows a faster forward motion.

Let your head lead the movement as you bring your right knee and left hand forwards simultaneously. Then let your left knee and right hand move forwards together. Continue this sequence, moving opposite knee and hand, while maintaining a long spine and relaxed breathing throughout.

# Simple cross-patterning

## 1/3 time

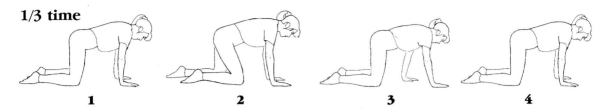

1. Start from the basic kneeling position, as before. (This is slightly more complicated than 1/4 time and 1/2 time, and is very close to the movement of a cantering horse.)

2. Let your head lead the movement as you allow your right knee to slide forward.

3. Then let your left knee and right hand move forward together.

4. Finally, your left hand moves forward, bringing you back to the starting position, ready to move forward once again.

Continue with this sequence. It may feel a little strange at first, but once you get into the rhythm it becomes much easier. Remember to keep your breathing relaxed and easy.

## Standing

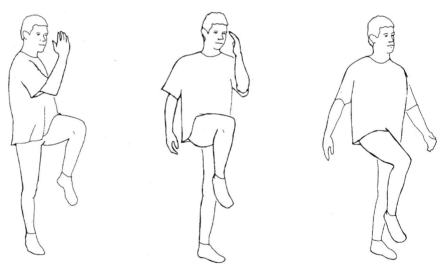

Begin by 'marking time' on the spot: lift each knee high in turn, bringing the opposite elbow across your body and towards your knee, in time with a natural marching rhythm. Exaggerate this movement, and continue for about one minute.

Now move into marking time in a normal marching movement, letting your arms swing in time with your legs: right arm swings forwards as left knee lifts, left arm swings forwards as right knee lifts.

Check that both arms swing an equal distance, forwards and back, and that you lift both knees to the same height.

# Summary

It will be apparent to students having worked through this book that the co-ordination patterns used here are but a few of the many hundreds that an imaginative mind could conceive. I am sure that, if you have understood the basic principles so far, most of you are now in a position to formulate and develop your own programmes, building on the ideas in the foregoing pages and incorporating them into everyday activities. Here are a few reminders of the basic principles:

- always aim to reduce effort, obtaining a relaxed, effortless action

- encourage natural functioning throughout your system by maintaining the working integrity of yourself as you move

- be aware of your own limitations, and always let yourself be guided by them in whatever you undertake

- expand your awareness to notice the joints and muscles involved in your movements

- enjoy the freedom of breathing easily, without strain

- let your face be relaxed and free of tension

- acquire a good sense of balance and poise, along with symmetrical development

- learn the ability to change your habitual manner of use of yourself when required

- understand that no aspect of yourself - physical, mental, emotional, psychological, spiritual - works in isolation. Each affects the rest

- always remember to keep your mind in the movement, your awareness in the action.

# Bibliography

Air Ministry: *Principles of Anatomy and Physiology for Physical Training Instructors, Royal Air Force,* HMSO, 1959.

Alexander, F. M.: *The Use of the Self,* Victor Gollancz, London, 1985, and *Constructive Conscious Control of the Individual,* Victor Gollancz, London, 1986.

Blaikie, William: *How to get strong and how to stay so,* Harper and Brothers, New York, 1879.

Checkley, Edwin: *A Natural Method of Physical Training,* William C. Bryant and Co., Brooklyn N.Y., 1890.

Devan, S. Arthur: *Exercise without Exercise,* Methuen and Co. Ltd., London, 1935.

Dunn, Beryl: *Dance Therapy for Dancers,* Heinemann Health Books, London, 1974.

Kapandji, I. A.: *The Physiology of the Joints,* Churchill Livingstone, Edinburgh, London and New York, 1970.

Michele, Arthur A.: *You don't have to ache,* Pan Books Ltd., London, 1972.

Pietroni, Patrick: *Holistic Living,* J. M.Dent and Sons Ltd., London and Melbourne, 1994.

Prabhavananda, Swami and Isherwood, Christopher: *How to know God, Yoga Aphorisms of Patanjali,* Cignet, New American Library, 1969.

Sheldon, W. H., *Varieties in Human Physique,* Harper, New York, 1940.

Svatmarama, *The Hatha Yoga Pradipika,* Adyar Library and Research Centre, 1972.

Truslow, Walter: *Body Poise,* Williams and Wilkins Co., Baltimore, 1943.

# Other publications from Bibliotek Books

**The Muscle Book** by Paul Blakey
Price £5.95 ISBN 1 873017 00 6

*"An inspired insight into the desire of the student for a clear and concise text on muscle anatomy."*
Ken Woodward FLCSP (Phys) Northern Institute of Massage.

**Stretching Without Pain** by Paul Blakey
Price £8.95 ISBN 1 873017 05 7

Clearly written and profusely illustrated to give you a thorough understanding of the principles of stretching. Every stretching method is explained so that you will be able to create your own training methods.

*Coming Soon...*

**Successful Fundraising** by John Baguley
ISBN 1 873017 15 4

A comprehensive and authorative handbook on the art of fundraising.

*Books may be ordered directly from Bibliotek Books. Send your order with a cheque made out to 'Bibliotek Books'. Discounts are given on orders of 10 or more. Please write for details.*

**Bibliotek Books**
**19 Warwick Road**
**Stafford ST17 4PD**